This book Belongs

To

. . . .

. . . .

How To Use The Book

- Tick or color the column $ for cash and C for card payments
- Choose the colors to represent spending choices (Necessary, Acceptable and Bad)

MONTH

Date	ITEM	$	C	Amount
	○			
	○			
	○			
	○			
	○			
	○			
	○			
	○			
	○			
	○			
	○			
	○			
	○			
	○			
	○			
	○			
	○			

○ Necessary   ○ Acceptable   ○ Bad   Total

MONTH

Date	ITEM	$	C	Amount

Necessary   Acceptable   Bad   Total

MONTH

Date		ITEM	$	C	Amount
	○				
	○				
	○				
	○				
	○				
	○				
	○				
	○				
	○				
	○				
	○				
	○				
	○				
	○				
	○				
	○				
	○				

○ Necessary   ○ Acceptable   ○ Bad   Total

MONTH

Date	ITEM	$	C	Amount

◯ Necessary ◯ Acceptable ◯ Bad   Total

MONTH

Date	ITEM	$	C	Amount
	○			
	○			
	○			
	○			
	○			
	○			
	○			
	○			
	○			
	○			
	○			
	○			
	○			
	○			
	○			
	○			
	○			

○ Necessary   ○ Acceptable   ○ Bad   Total

MONTH

Date	ITEM	$	C	Amount
	◯			
	◯			
	◯			
	◯			
	◯			
	◯			
	◯			
	◯			
	◯			
	◯			
	◯			
	◯			
	◯			
	◯			
	◯			
	◯			
	◯			

◯ Necessary   ◯ Acceptable   ◯ Bad   Total

MONTH

Date	ITEM	$	C	Amount
	⚪			
	⚪			
	⚪			
	⚪			
	⚪			
	⚪			
	⚪			
	⚪			
	⚪			
	⚪			
	⚪			
	⚪			
	⚪			
	⚪			
	⚪			
	⚪			

⚪ Necessary   ⚪ Acceptable   ⚪ Bad   Total

MONTH

Date	ITEM	$	C	Amount

○ Necessary   ○ Acceptable   ○ Bad   Total

MONTH

Date		ITEM	$	C	Amount
	○				
	○				
	○				
	○				
	○				
	○				
	○				
	○				
	○				
	○				
	○				
	○				
	○				
	○				
	○				
	○				
	○				

○ Necessary   ○ Acceptable   ○ Bad   Total

MONTH

Date	ITEM	$	C	Amount

Necessary　　Acceptable　　Bad　　Total

MONTH

Date	ITEM	$	C	Amount
	○			
	○			
	○			
	○			
	○			
	○			
	○			
	○			
	○			
	○			
	○			
	○			
	○			
	○			
	○			
	○			
	○			

○ Necessary   ○ Acceptable   ○ Bad   Total

MONTH

Date	ITEM	$	C	Amount
	○			
	○			
	○			
	○			
	○			
	○			
	○			
	○			
	○			
	○			
	○			
	○			
	○			
	○			
	○			
	○			
	○			

○ Necessary   ○ Acceptable   ○ Bad   Total

MONTH

Date		ITEM	$	C	Amount
	○				
	○				
	○				
	○				
	○				
	○				
	○				
	○				
	○				
	○				
	○				
	○				
	○				
	○				
	○		$	C	
	○				
	○				

○ Necessary   ○ Acceptable   ○ Bad   Total

MONTH

Date	ITEM	$	C	Amount

Necessary   Acceptable   Bad   Total

Date		ITEM	$	C	Amount
	○				
	○				
	○				
	○				
	○				
	○				
	○				
	○				
	○				
	○				
	○				
	○				
	○				
	○				
	○				
	○				
	○				

MONTH

○ Necessary   ○ Acceptable   ○ Bad   Total

MONTH

Date	ITEM	$	C	Amount

Necessary   Acceptable   Bad   Total

MONTH

Date	ITEM	$	C	Amount
	○			
	○			
	○			
	○			
	○			
	○			
	○			
	○			
	○			
	○			
	○			
	○			
	○			
	○			
	○			
	○			
	○			

○ Necessary　　○ Acceptable　　○ Bad　　Total

MONTH

Date	ITEM	$	C	Amount
	○			
	○			
	○			
	○			
	○			
	○			
	○			
	○			
	○			
	○			
	○			
	○			
	○			
	○			
	○			
	○			
	○			

○ Necessary   ○ Acceptable   ○ Bad   Total

MONTH

Date	ITEM	$	C	Amount
	◯			
	◯			
	◯			
	◯			
	◯			
	◯			
	◯			
	◯			
	◯			
	◯			
	◯			
	◯			
	◯			
	◯			
	◯			
	◯			

◯ Necessary　　◯ Acceptable　　◯ Bad　　Total

MONTH

Date	ITEM	$	C	Amount

Necessary   Acceptable   Bad   Total

MONTH

Date		ITEM	$	C	Amount
	○				
	○				
	○				
	○				
	○				
	○				
	○				
	○				
	○				
	○				
	○				
	○				
	○				
	○				
	○				
	○				

○ Necessary   ○ Acceptable   ○ Bad   Total

MONTH

Date	ITEM	$	C	Amount

○ Necessary　　○ Acceptable　　○ Bad　　Total

MONTH

Date	ITEM	$	C	Amount
	○			
	○			
	○			
	○			
	○			
	○			
	○			
	○			
	○			
	○			
	○			
	○			
	○			
	○			
	○			
	○			
	○			

○ Necessary   ○ Acceptable   ○ Bad   Total

MONTH

Date	ITEM	$	C	Amount
	○			
	○			
	○			
	○			
	○			
	○			
	○			
	○			
	○			
	○			
	○			
	○			
	○			
	○			
	○			
	○			
	○			

○ Necessary   ○ Acceptable   ○ Bad   Total

MONTH

Date		ITEM	$	C	Amount
	○				
	○				
	○				
	○				
	○				
	○				
	○				
	○				
	○				
	○				
	○				
	○				
	○				
	○				
	○				
	○				
	○				

○ Necessary   ○ **Acceptable**   ○ Bad   Total

MONTH

Date	ITEM	$	C	Amount

Necessary   Acceptable   Bad   Total

MONTH

Date		ITEM	$	C	Amount
	○				
	○				
	○				
	○				
	○				
	○				
	○				
	○				
	○				
	○				
	○				
	○				
	○				
	○				
	○				
	○				
	○				

○ Necessary   ○ Acceptable   ○ Bad   Total

MONTH

Date	ITEM	$	C	Amount

Necessary   Acceptable   Bad   Total

MONTH

Date	ITEM	$	C	Amount
	○			
	○			
	○			
	○			
	○			
	○			
	○			
	○			
	○			
	○			
	○			
	○			
	○			
	○			
	○			
	○			
	○			

○ Necessary   ○ Acceptable   ○ Bad   Total

MONTH

Date	ITEM	$	C	Amount
	○			
	○			
	○			
	○			
	○			
	○			
	○			
	○			
	○			
	○			
	○			
	○			
	○			
	○			
	○			
	○			
	○			

○ Necessary   ○ Acceptable   ○ Bad   Total [   ]

MONTH

Date	ITEM	$	C	Amount
	○			
	○			
	○			
	○			
	○			
	○			
	○			
	○			
	○			
	○			
	○			
	○			
	○			
	○			
	○			
	○			
	○			

○ Necessary   ○ Acceptable   ○ Bad   Total

MONTH

Date	ITEM	$	C	Amount

Necessary   Acceptable   Bad   Total

MONTH

Date		ITEM	$	C	Amount
	○				
	○				
	○				
	○				
	○				
	○				
	○				
	○				
	○				
	○				
	○				
	○				
	○				
	○				
	○				
	○				
	○				

○ Necessary   ○ Acceptable   ○ Bad   Total

MONTH

Date	ITEM	$	C	Amount

Necessary   Acceptable   Bad   Total

MONTH

Date	ITEM	$	C	Amount
	○			
	○			
	○			
	○			
	○			
	○			
	○			
	○			
	○			
	○			
	○			
	○			
	○			
	○			
	○			
	○			
	○			

○ Necessary   ○ Acceptable   ○ Bad   Total

MONTH

Date	ITEM	$	C	Amount

○ Necessary   ○ Acceptable   ○ Bad   Total

MONTH

Date	ITEM	$	C	Amount
	○			
	○			
	○			
	○			
	○			
	○			
	○			
	○			
	○			
	○			
	○			
	○			
	○			
	○			
	○			
	○			
	○			

○ Necessary   ○ Acceptable   ○ Bad   Total

MONTH

Date	ITEM	$	C	Amount

Necessary   Acceptable   Bad   Total

MONTH

Date		ITEM	$	C	Amount
	○				
	○				
	○				
	○				
	○				
	○				
	○				
	○				
	○				
	○				
	○				
	○				
	○				
	○				
	○				
	○				
	○				

○ Necessary   ○ Acceptable   ○ Bad   Total

MONTH

Date	ITEM	$	C	Amount

Necessary   Acceptable   Bad   Total

MONTH

Date		ITEM	$	C	Amount
	○				
	○				
	○				
	○				
	○				
	○				
	○				
	○				
	○				
	○				
	○				
	○				
	○				
	○				
	○				
	○				
	○				

○ Necessary   ○ Acceptable   ○ Bad   Total

MONTH

Date	ITEM	$	C	Amount

○ Necessary   ○ Acceptable   ○ Bad   Total

MONTH

Date		ITEM	$	C	Amount
	○				
	○				
	○				
	○				
	○				
	○				
	○				
	○				
	○				
	○				
	○				
	○				
	○				
	○				
	○				
	○				
	○				

○ Necessary   ○ Acceptable   ○ Bad   Total

MONTH

Date	ITEM	$	C	Amount

○ Necessary   ○ Acceptable   ○ Bad   Total

MONTH

Date		ITEM	$	C	Amount
	○				
	○				
	○				
	○				
	○				
	○				
	○				
	○				
	○				
	○				
	○				
	○				
	○				
	○				
	○				
	○				
	○				

○ Necessary   ○ Acceptable   ○ Bad   Total

MONTH

Date	ITEM	$	C	Amount

Necessary   Acceptable   Bad   Total

MONTH

Date	ITEM	$	C	Amount
	○			
	○			
	○			
	○			
	○			
	○			
	○			
	○			
	○			
	○			
	○			
	○			
	○			
	○			
	○			
	○			
	○			

○ Necessary   ○ Acceptable   ○ Bad   Total

MONTH

Date	ITEM	$	C	Amount
	○			
	○			
	○			
	○			
	○			
	○			
	○			
	○			
	○			
	○			
	○			
	○			
	○			
	○			
	○			
	○			
	○			

○ Necessary　　○ Acceptable　　○ Bad　　Total

MONTH

Date	ITEM	$	C	Amount
	○			
	○			
	○			
	○			
	○			
	○			
	○			
	○			
	○			
	○			
	○			
	○			
	○			
	○			
	○			
	○			
	○			

○ Necessary   ○ Acceptable   ○ Bad   Total

MONTH

Date	ITEM	$	C	Amount

◯ Necessary   ◯ Acceptable   ◯ Bad   Total

MONTH

Date		ITEM	$	C	Amount
	○				
	○				
	○				
	○				
	○				
	○				
	○				
	○				
	○				
	○				
	○				
	○				
	○				
	○				
	○				
	○				
	○				

○ Necessary   ○ Acceptable   ○ Bad   Total

MONTH

Date	ITEM	$	C	Amount

Necessary   Acceptable   Bad   Total

MONTH

Date	ITEM	$	C	Amount
	○			
	○			
	○			
	○			
	○			
	○			
	○			
	○			
	○			
	○			
	○			
	○			
	○			
	○			
	○			
	○			
	○			

○ Necessary   ○ Acceptable   ○ Bad   Total

MONTH

Date	ITEM	$	C	Amount
	○			
	○			
	○			
	○			
	○			
	○			
	○			
	○			
	○			
	○			
	○			
	○			
	○			
	○			
	○			
	○			
	○			

○ Necessary ○ Acceptable ○ Bad Total

MONTH

Date	ITEM	$	C	Amount
	○			
	○			
	○			
	○			
	○			
	○			
	○			
	○			
	○			
	○			
	○			
	○			
	○			
	○			
	○			
	○			
	○			

○ Necessary   ○ Acceptable   ○ Bad   Total

MONTH

Date	ITEM	$	C	Amount

Necessary   Acceptable   Bad   Total

MONTH

Date		ITEM	$	C	Amount
	○				
	○				
	○				
	○				
	○				
	○				
	○				
	○				
	○				
	○				
	○				
	○				
	○				
	○				
	○				
	○				
	○				

○ Necessary   ○ Acceptable   ○ Bad   Total

MONTH

Date	ITEM	$	C	Amount

◯ Necessary ◯ Acceptable ◯ Bad Total

MONTH

Date		ITEM	$	C	Amount
	○				
	○				
	○				
	○				
	○				
	○				
	○				
	○				
	○				
	○				
	○				
	○				
	○				
	○				
	○				
	○				
	○				

○ Necessary   ○ Acceptable   ○ Bad   Total

MONTH

Date	ITEM	$	C	Amount
	○			
	○			
	○			
	○			
	○			
	○			
	○			
	○			
	○			
	○			
	○			
	○			
	○			
	○			
	○			
	○			
	○			

○ Necessary   ○ Acceptable   ○ Bad   Total

MONTH

Date	ITEM	$	C	Amount
	○			
	○			
	○			
	○			
	○			
	○			
	○			
	○			
	○			
	○			
	○			
	○			
	○			
	○			
	○			
	○			
	○			

○ Necessary   ○ Acceptable   ○ Bad   Total

MONTH

Date	ITEM	$	C	Amount

○ Necessary   ○ Acceptable   ○ Bad   Total

MONTH

Date	ITEM	$	C	Amount
	⚪			
	⚪			
	⚪			
	⚪			
	⚪			
	⚪			
	⚪			
	⚪			
	⚪			
	⚪			
	⚪			
	⚪			
	⚪			
	⚪			
	⚪			
	⚪			
	⚪			

⚪ Necessary   ⚪ Acceptable   ⚪ Bad   Total

MONTH

Date	ITEM	$	C	Amount

Necessary   Acceptable   Bad   Total

MONTH

Date		ITEM	$	C	Amount
	○				
	○				
	○				
	○				
	○				
	○				
	○				
	○				
	○				
	○				
	○				
	○				
	○				
	○				
	○				
	○				
	○				

○ Necessary   ○ Acceptable   ○ Bad   Total

MONTH

Date	ITEM	$	C	Amount

○ Necessary   ○ Acceptable   ○ Bad   Total

MONTH

Date		ITEM	$	C	Amount
	○				
	○				
	○				
	○				
	○				
	○				
	○				
	○				
	○				
	○				
	○				
	○				
	○				
	○				
	○				
	○				
	○				

○ Necessary   ○ Acceptable   ○ Bad   Total

MONTH

Date	ITEM	$	C	Amount

○ Necessary   ○ Acceptable   ○ Bad   Total

MONTH

Date		ITEM	$	C	Amount
	○				
	○				
	○				
	○				
	○				
	○				
	○				
	○				
	○				
	○				
	○				
	○				
	○				
	○				
	○				
	○				
	○				

○ Necessary   ○ Acceptable   ○ Bad   Total

MONTH

Date	ITEM	$	C	Amount

Necessary   Acceptable   Bad   Total

MONTH

Date	ITEM	$	C	Amount
	○			
	○			
	○			
	○			
	○			
	○			
	○			
	○			
	○			
	○			
	○			
	○			
	○			
	○			
	○			
	○			
	○			

○ Necessary   ○ Acceptable   ○ Bad   Total

MONTH

Date	ITEM	$	C	Amount

○ Necessary   ○ Acceptable   ○ Bad   Total

MONTH

Date	ITEM	$	C	Amount
	○			
	○			
	○			
	○			
	○			
	○			
	○			
	○			
	○			
	○			
	○			
	○			
	○			
	○			
	○			
	○			
	○			

○ Necessary   ○ Acceptable   ○ Bad   Total

MONTH

Date	ITEM	$	C	Amount

◯ Necessary   ◯ Acceptable   ◯ Bad   Total

MONTH

Date	ITEM	$	C	Amount
	○			
	○			
	○			
	○			
	○			
	○			
	○			
	○			
	○			
	○			
	○			
	○			
	○			
	○			
	○			
	○			
	○			

○ Necessary   ○ Acceptable   ○ Bad   Total

MONTH

Date	ITEM	$	C	Amount

○ Necessary   ○ Acceptable   ○ Bad   Total

MONTH

Date		ITEM	$	C	Amount
	○				
	○				
	○				
	○				
	○				
	○				
	○				
	○				
	○				
	○				
	○				
	○				
	○				
	○				
	○				
	○				
	○				

○ Necessary   ○ Acceptable   ○ Bad   Total

MONTH

Date	ITEM	$	C	Amount

○ Necessary   ○ Acceptable   ○ Bad   Total

MONTH

Date	ITEM	$	C	Amount
	○			
	○			
	○			
	○			
	○			
	○			
	○			
	○			
	○			
	○			
	○			
	○			
	○			
	○			
	○			
	○			
	○			

○ Necessary   ○ Acceptable   ○ Bad   Total

MONTH

Date	ITEM	$	C	Amount

Necessary   Acceptable   Bad   Total

MONTH

Date	ITEM	$	C	Amount
	○			
	○			
	○			
	○			
	○			
	○			
	○			
	○			
	○			
	○			
	○			
	○			
	○			
	○			
	○			
	○			
	○			

○ Necessary   ○ Acceptable   ○ Bad   Total

MONTH

Date	ITEM	$	C	Amount

○ Necessary   ○ Acceptable   ○ Bad   Total

MONTH

Date		ITEM	$	C	Amount
	○				
	○				
	○				
	○				
	○				
	○				
	○				
	○				
	○				
	○				
	○				
	○				
	○				
	○				
	○				
	○				
	○				

○ Necessary　　　○ Acceptable　　　○ Bad　　　Total

MONTH

Date	ITEM	$	C	Amount

○ Necessary   ○ Acceptable   ○ Bad   Total

MONTH

Date	ITEM	$	C	Amount
	○			
	○			
	○			
	○			
	○			
	○			
	○			
	○			
	○			
	○			
	○			
	○			
	○			
	○			
	○			
	○			
	○			

○ Necessary   ○ Acceptable   ○ Bad   Total

MONTH

Date	ITEM	$	C	Amount

○ Necessary   ○ Acceptable   ○ Bad   Total

MONTH

Date		ITEM	$	C	Amount
	⭕				
	⭕				
	⭕				
	⭕				
	⭕				
	⭕				
	⭕				
	⭕				
	⭕				
	⭕				
	⭕				
	⭕				
	⭕				
	⭕				
	⭕				
	⭕				

⭕ Necessary ⭕ Acceptable ⭕ Bad Total

MONTH

Date	ITEM	$	C	Amount

○ Necessary   ○ Acceptable   ○ Bad   Total

MONTH

Date		ITEM	$	C	Amount
	○				
	○				
	○				
	○				
	○				
	○				
	○				
	○				
	○				
	○				
	○				
	○				
	○				
	○				
	○				
	○				
	○				

○ Necessary   ○ Acceptable   ○ Bad   Total

MONTH

Date	ITEM	$	C	Amount

◯ Necessary   ◯ Acceptable   ◯ Bad   Total

MONTH

Date		ITEM	$	C	Amount
	◯				
	◯				
	◯				
	◯				
	◯				
	◯				
	◯				
	◯				
	◯				
	◯				
	◯				
	◯				
	◯				
	◯				
	◯				
	◯				
	◯				

◯ Necessary   ◯ Acceptable   ◯ Bad   Total

MONTH

Date	ITEM	$	C	Amount

○ Necessary   ○ Acceptable   ○ Bad   Total

MONTH

Date	ITEM	$	C	Amount
	○			
	○			
	○			
	○			
	○			
	○			
	○			
	○			
	○			
	○			
	○			
	○			
	○			
	○			
	○			
	○			
	○			

○ Necessary   ○ Acceptable   ○ Bad   Total

MONTH

Date	ITEM	$	C	Amount

◯ Necessary   ◯ Acceptable   ◯ Bad   Total [   ]

MONTH

Date	ITEM	$	C	Amount
	○			
	○			
	○			
	○			
	○			
	○			
	○			
	○			
	○			
	○			
	○			
	○			
	○			
	○			
	○			
	○			
	○			

○ Necessary   ○ Acceptable   ○ Bad   Total

MONTH

Date	ITEM	$	C	Amount
	○			
	○			
	○			
	○			
	○			
	○			
	○			
	○			
	○			
	○			
	○			
	○			
	○			
	○			
	○			
	○			
	○			

○ Necessary   ○ Acceptable   ○ Bad   Total

MONTH

Date	ITEM	$	C	Amount
	○			
	○			
	○			
	○			
	○			
	○			
	○			
	○			
	○			
	○			
	○			
	○			
	○			
	○			
	○			
	○			

○ Necessary ○ Acceptable ○ Bad Total

MONTH

Date	ITEM	$	C	Amount

○ Necessary   ○ Acceptable   ○ Bad   Total

MONTH

Date		ITEM	$	C	Amount
	○				
	○				
	○				
	○				
	○				
	○				
	○				
	○				
	○				
	○				
	○				
	○				
	○				
	○				
	○				
	○				

○ Necessary   ○ Acceptable   ○ Bad   Total

Made in United States
North Haven, CT
27 September 2023

42046380R00055